AF371356

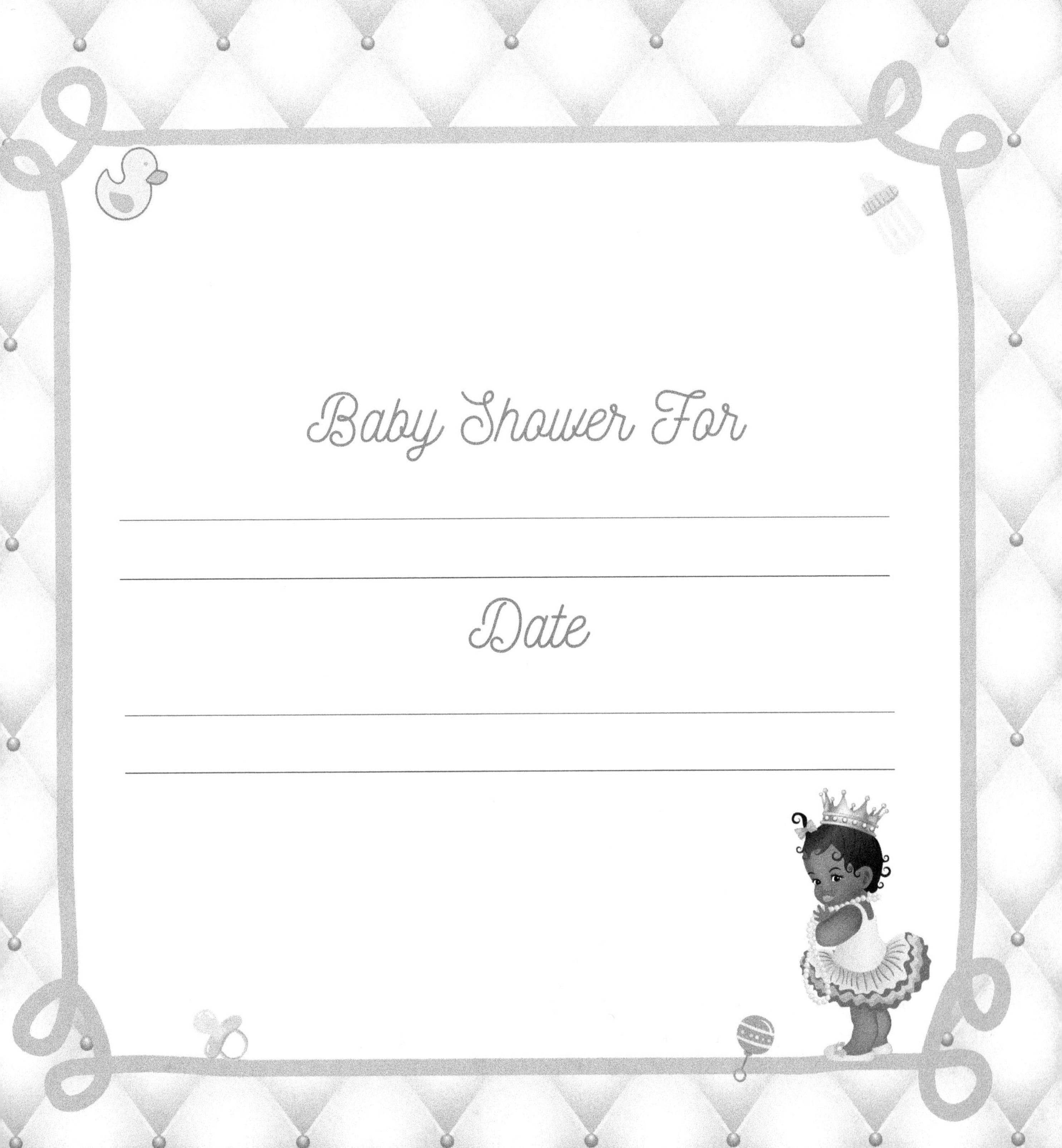

Baby Shower For
Date

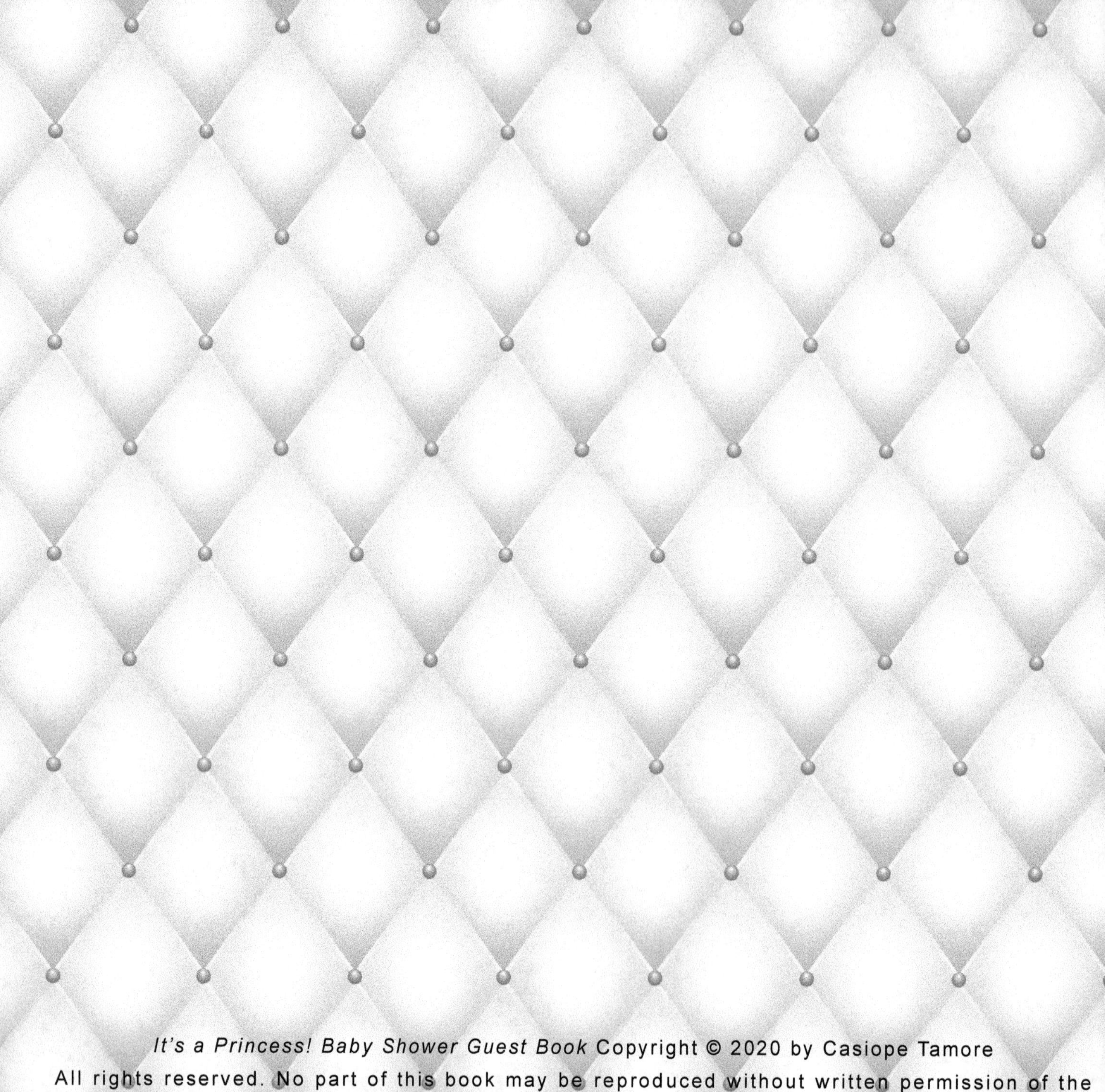

Guest Name

Relationship to Parents

Advice for Parents

Wishes for Baby

Guest Name

Relationship to Parents

Advice for Parents

Wishes for Baby

Guest Name

____

Relationship to Parents

____

Advice for Parents

____

____

____

Wishes for Baby

____

____

____

Guest Name

____

Relationship to Parents

____

Advice for Parents

____

____

____

____

Wishes for Baby

____

____

____

____

Guest Name

____

Relationship to Parents

____

Advice for Parents

____

____

____

Wishes for Baby

____

____

____

Guest Name

____

Relationship to Parents

____

Advice for Parents

____

____

____

____

Wishes for Baby

____

____

____

____

Guest Name

Relationship to Parents

Advice for Parents

Wishes for Baby

Guest Name

Relationship to Parents

Advice for Parents

Wishes for Baby

Guest Name

Relationship to Parents

Advice for Parents

Wishes for Baby

Guest Name

Relationship to Parents

Advice for Parents

Wishes for Baby

Guest Name

Relationship to Parents

Advice for Parents

Wishes for Baby

Guest Name

Relationship to Parents

Advice for Parents

Wishes for Baby

Guest Name

Relationship to Parents

Advice for Parents

Wishes for Baby

Guest Name

Relationship to Parents

Advice for Parents

Wishes for Baby

Guest Name

Relationship to Parents

Advice for Parents

Wishes for Baby

Guest Name

____

Relationship to Parents

____

Advice for Parents

____

____

____

____

Wishes for Baby

____

____

____

Guest Name

Relationship to Parents

Advice for Parents

Wishes for Baby

Guest Name

Relationship to Parents

Advice for Parents

Wishes for Baby

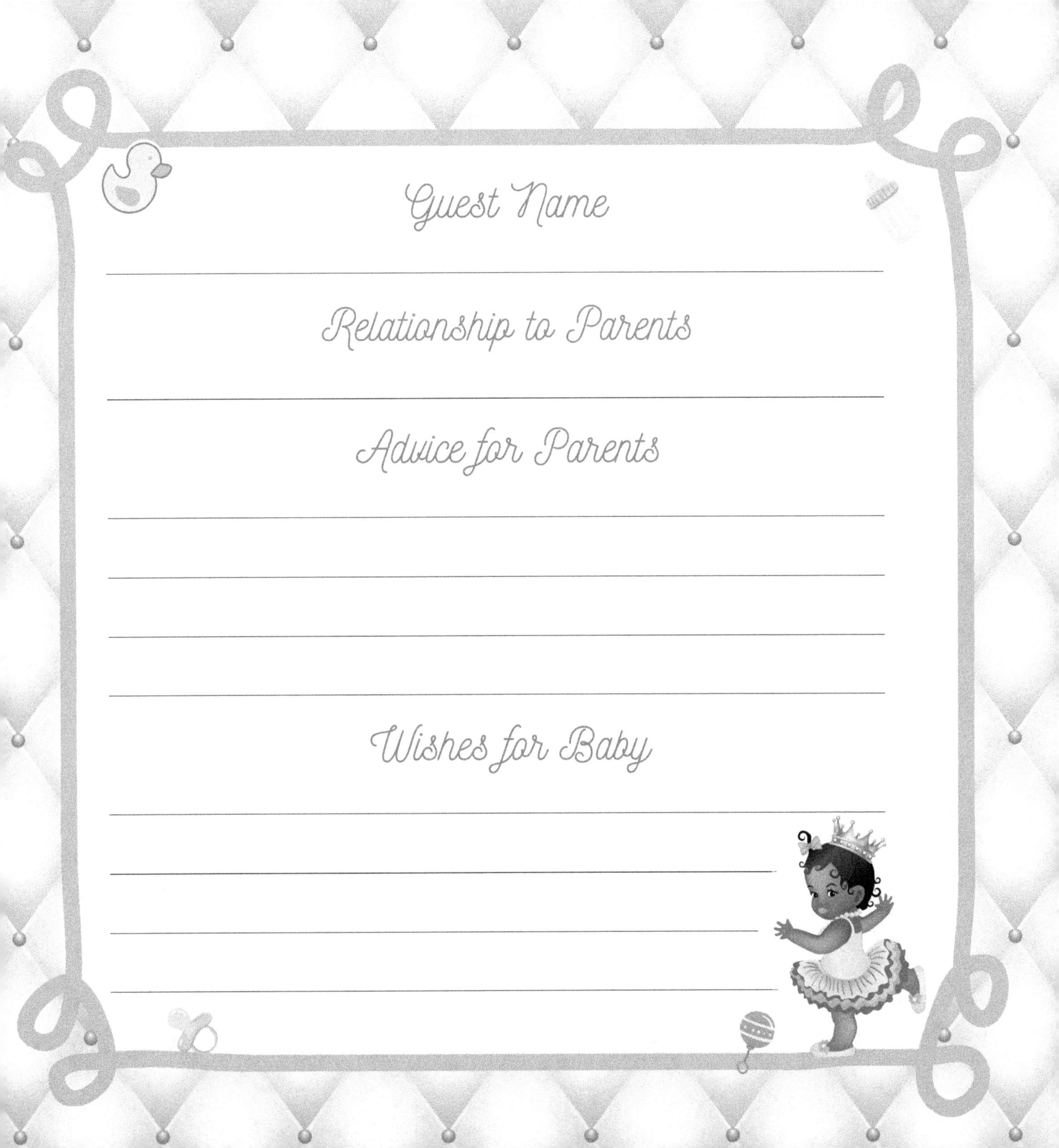

Guest Name

Relationship to Parents

Advice for Parents

Wishes for Baby

Guest Name

Relationship to Parents

Advice for Parents

Wishes for Baby

Guest Name

Relationship to Parents

Advice for Parents

Wishes for Baby

Guest Name

Relationship to Parents

Advice for Parents

Wishes for Baby

Guest Name

Relationship to Parents

Advice for Parents

Wishes for Baby

Guest Name

Relationship to Parents

Advice for Parents

Wishes for Baby

Guest Name

Relationship to Parents

Advice for Parents

Wishes for Baby

Guest Name

Relationship to Parents

Advice for Parents

Wishes for Baby

Guest Name

Relationship to Parents

Advice for Parents

Wishes for Baby

Guest Name

Relationship to Parents

Advice for Parents

Wishes for Baby

Guest Name

Relationship to Parents

Advice for Parents

Wishes for Baby

Guest Name

Relationship to Parents

Advice for Parents

Wishes for Baby

Guest Name

Relationship to Parents

Advice for Parents

Wishes for Baby

Guest Name

Relationship to Parents

Advice for Parents

Wishes for Baby

Guest Name

____

Relationship to Parents

____

Advice for Parents

____

____

____

Wishes for Baby

____

____

____

Guest Name

____

Relationship to Parents

____

Advice for Parents

____

____

____

Wishes for Baby

____

____

____

Guest Name

Relationship to Parents

Advice for Parents

Wishes for Baby

Guest Name

Relationship to Parents

Advice for Parents

Wishes for Baby

Guest Name

Relationship to Parents

Advice for Parents

Wishes for Baby

Guest Name

Relationship to Parents

Advice for Parents

Wishes for Baby

Guest Name

Relationship to Parents

Advice for Parents

Wishes for Baby

Guest Name

Relationship to Parents

Advice for Parents

Wishes for Baby

Guest Name

Relationship to Parents

Advice for Parents

Wishes for Baby

Guest Name

____

Relationship to Parents

____

Advice for Parents

____

____

____

Wishes for Baby

____

____

____

Guest Name

Relationship to Parents

Advice for Parents

Wishes for Baby

Guest Name

Relationship to Parents

Advice for Parents

Wishes for Baby

Guest Name

Relationship to Parents

Advice for Parents

Wishes for Baby

Guest Name

Relationship to Parents

Advice for Parents

Wishes for Baby

Guest Name

Relationship to Parents

Advice for Parents

Wishes for Baby

Guest Name

Relationship to Parents

Advice for Parents

Wishes for Baby

Guest Name

Relationship to Parents

Advice for Parents

Wishes for Baby

Guest Name

Relationship to Parents

Advice for Parents

Wishes for Baby

Guest Name

____

Relationship to Parents

____

Advice for Parents

____

____

____

____

Wishes for Baby

____

____

____

Guest Name

Relationship to Parents

Advice for Parents

Wishes for Baby

Guest Name

Relationship to Parents

Advice for Parents

Wishes for Baby

Guest Name

Relationship to Parents

Advice for Parents

Wishes for Baby

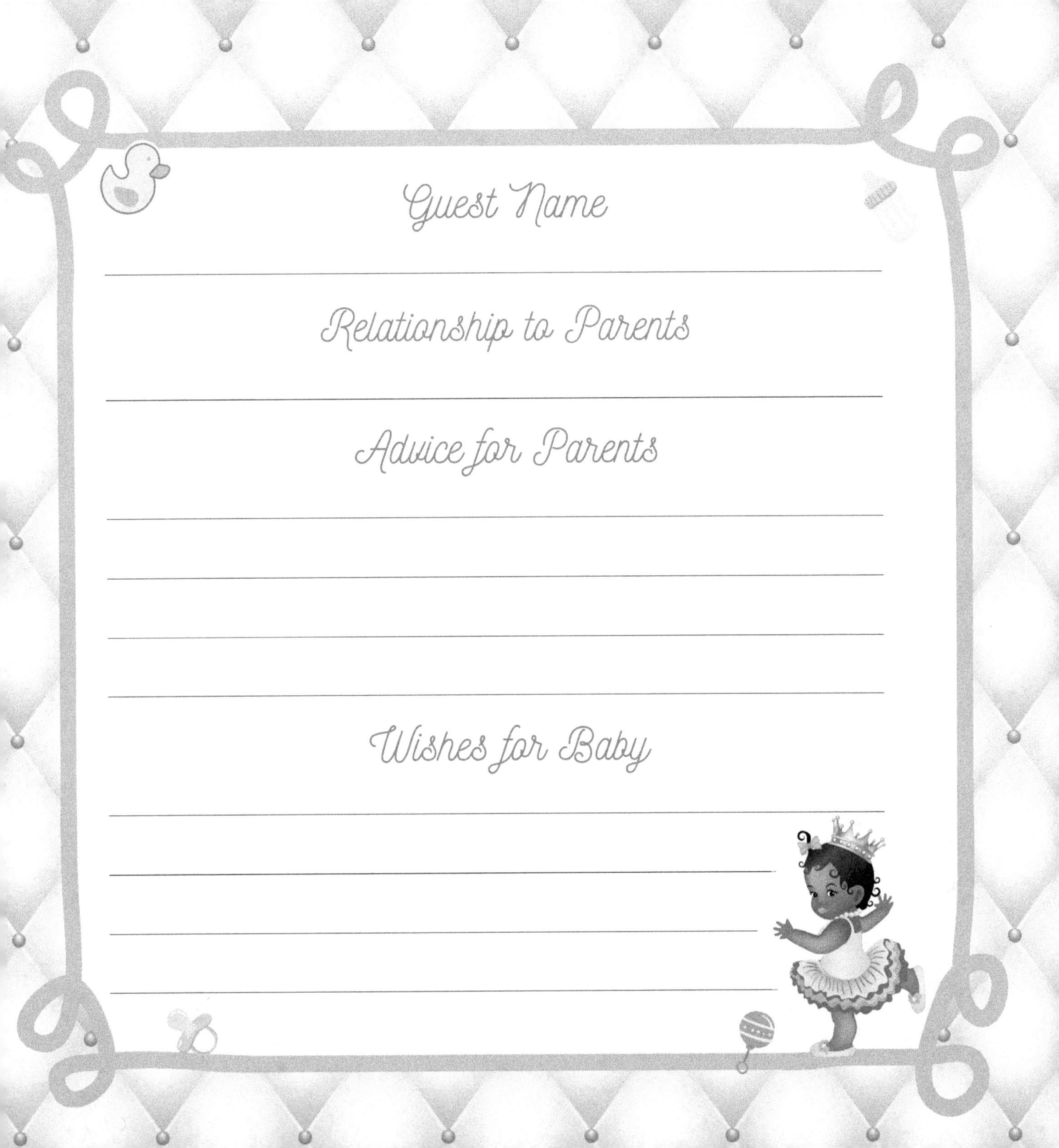

Guest Name

Relationship to Parents

Advice for Parents

Wishes for Baby

Guest Name

Relationship to Parents

Advice for Parents

Wishes for Baby

Guest Name

Relationship to Parents

Advice for Parents

Wishes for Baby

Guest Name

Relationship to Parents

Advice for Parents

Wishes for Baby

Guest Name

Relationship to Parents

Advice for Parents

Wishes for Baby

Guest Name

____

Relationship to Parents

____

Advice for Parents

____

____

____

Wishes for Baby

____

____

____

Guest Name

Relationship to Parents

Advice for Parents

Wishes for Baby

Guest Name

____

Relationship to Parents

____

Advice for Parents

____

____

____

____

Wishes for Baby

____

____

____

____

Guest Name

Relationship to Parents

Advice for Parents

Wishes for Baby

Guest Name

____

Relationship to Parents

____

Advice for Parents

____

____

____

____

Wishes for Baby

____

____

____

Guest Name

Relationship to Parents

Advice for Parents

Wishes for Baby

Guest Name

____

Relationship to Parents

____

Advice for Parents

____

____

____

____

Wishes for Baby

____

____

____

Guest Name

Relationship to Parents

Advice for Parents

Wishes for Baby

Guest Name

Relationship to Parents

Advice for Parents

Wishes for Baby

Guest Name

____

Relationship to Parents

____

Advice for Parents

____

____

____

Wishes for Baby

____

____

____

Guest Name

Relationship to Parents

Advice for Parents

Wishes for Baby

Guest Name

Relationship to Parents

Advice for Parents

Wishes for Baby

Guest Name

Relationship to Parents

Advice for Parents

Wishes for Baby

Guest Name

____

Relationship to Parents

____

Advice for Parents

____

____

____

____

Wishes for Baby

____

____

____

Guest Name

____

Relationship to Parents

____

Advice for Parents

____

____

____

Wishes for Baby

____

____

____

Guest Name

Relationship to Parents

Advice for Parents

Wishes for Baby

Guest Name

____

Relationship to Parents

____

Advice for Parents

____

____

____

Wishes for Baby

____

____

____

Guest Name

Relationship to Parents

Advice for Parents

Wishes for Baby

Guest Name

Relationship to Parents

Advice for Parents

Wishes for Baby

Guest Name

Relationship to Parents

Advice for Parents

Wishes for Baby

Guest Name

Relationship to Parents

Advice for Parents

Wishes for Baby

Guest Name

Relationship to Parents

Advice for Parents

Wishes for Baby

Guest Name

____

Relationship to Parents

____

Advice for Parents

____

____

____

____

Wishes for Baby

____

____

____

Guest Name

Relationship to Parents

Advice for Parents

Wishes for Baby

Guest Name

Relationship to Parents

Advice for Parents

Wishes for Baby

Guest Name

Relationship to Parents

Advice for Parents

Wishes for Baby

Guest Name

Relationship to Parents

Advice for Parents

Wishes for Baby

Guest Name

Relationship to Parents

Advice for Parents

Wishes for Baby

Guest Name

Relationship to Parents

Advice for Parents

Wishes for Baby

Guest Name

Relationship to Parents

Advice for Parents

Wishes for Baby

Guest Name

____

Relationship to Parents

____

Advice for Parents

____

____

____

Wishes for Baby

____

____

____

Guest Name

Relationship to Parents

Advice for Parents

Wishes for Baby

Guest Name

Relationship to Parents

Advice for Parents

Wishes for Baby

Guest Name

Relationship to Parents

Advice for Parents

Wishes for Baby

Guest Name

Relationship to Parents

Advice for Parents

Wishes for Baby

Guest Name

Relationship to Parents

Advice for Parents

Wishes for Baby

Guest Name

Relationship to Parents

Advice for Parents

Wishes for Baby

Guest Name

Relationship to Parents

Advice for Parents

Wishes for Baby

Guest Name

Relationship to Parents

Advice for Parents

Wishes for Baby

Guest Name

Relationship to Parents

Advice for Parents

Wishes for Baby

Guest Name

____

Relationship to Parents

____

Advice for Parents

____

____

____

Wishes for Baby

____

____

____

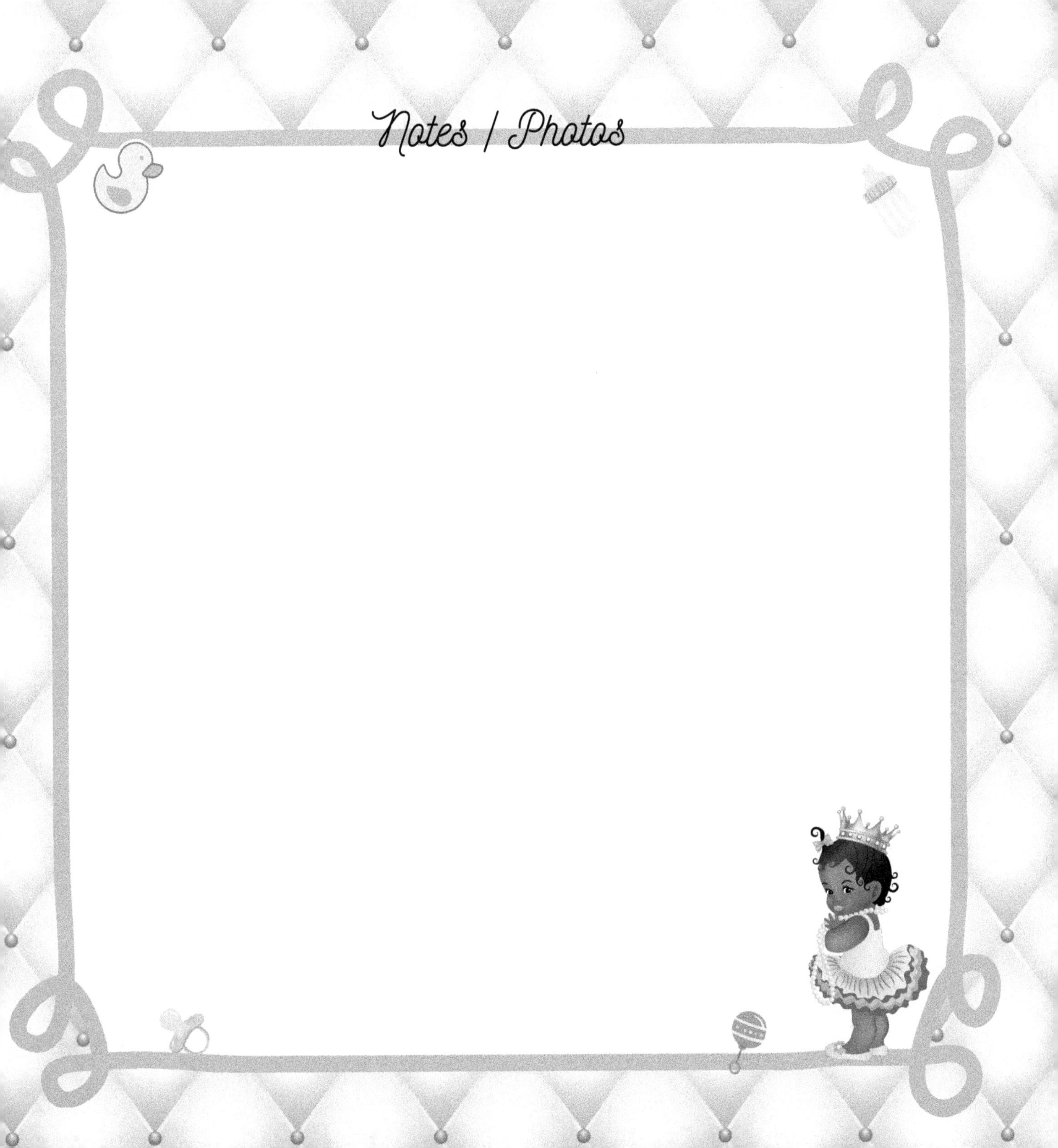

Notes / Photos

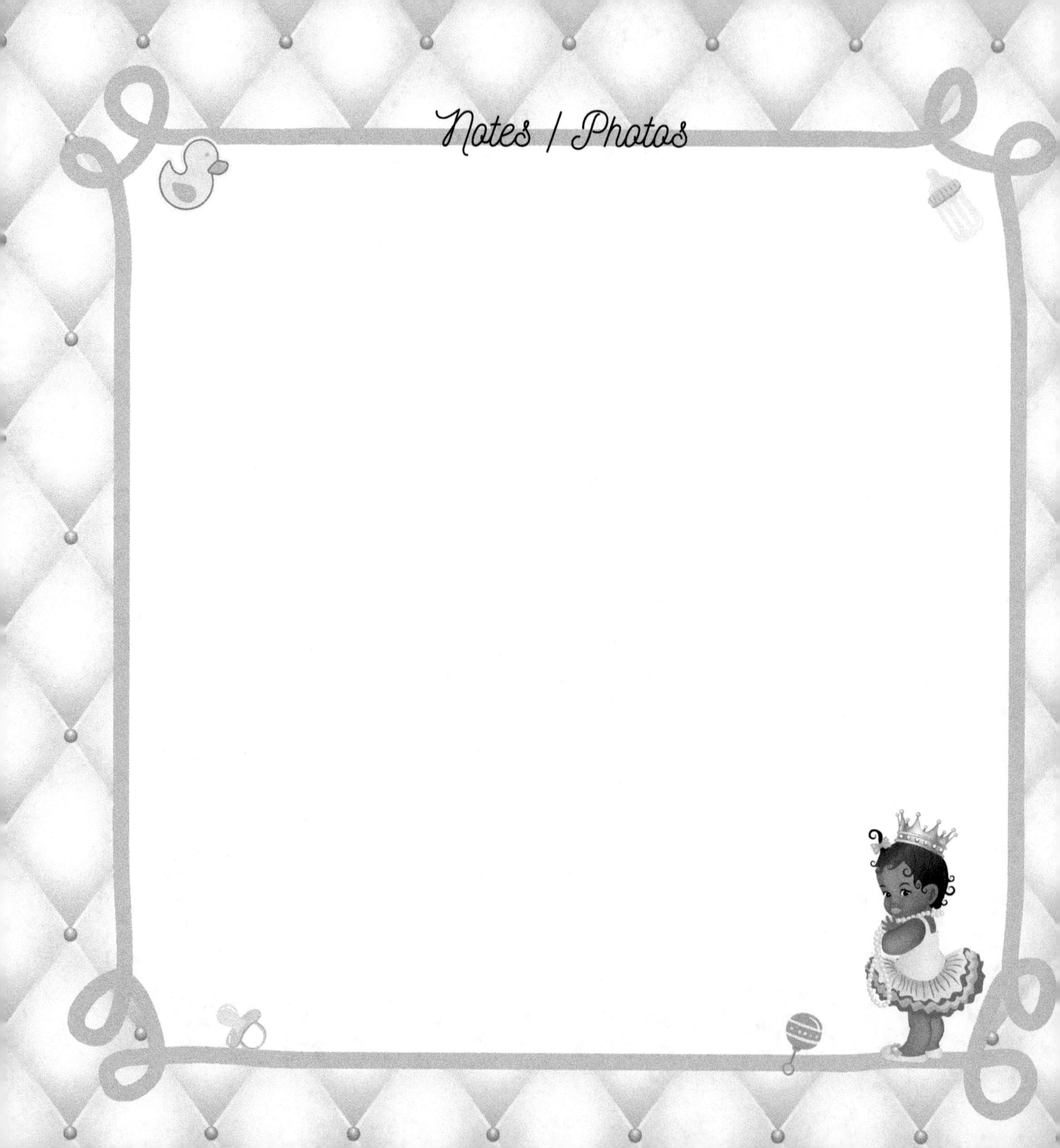

Notes / Photos

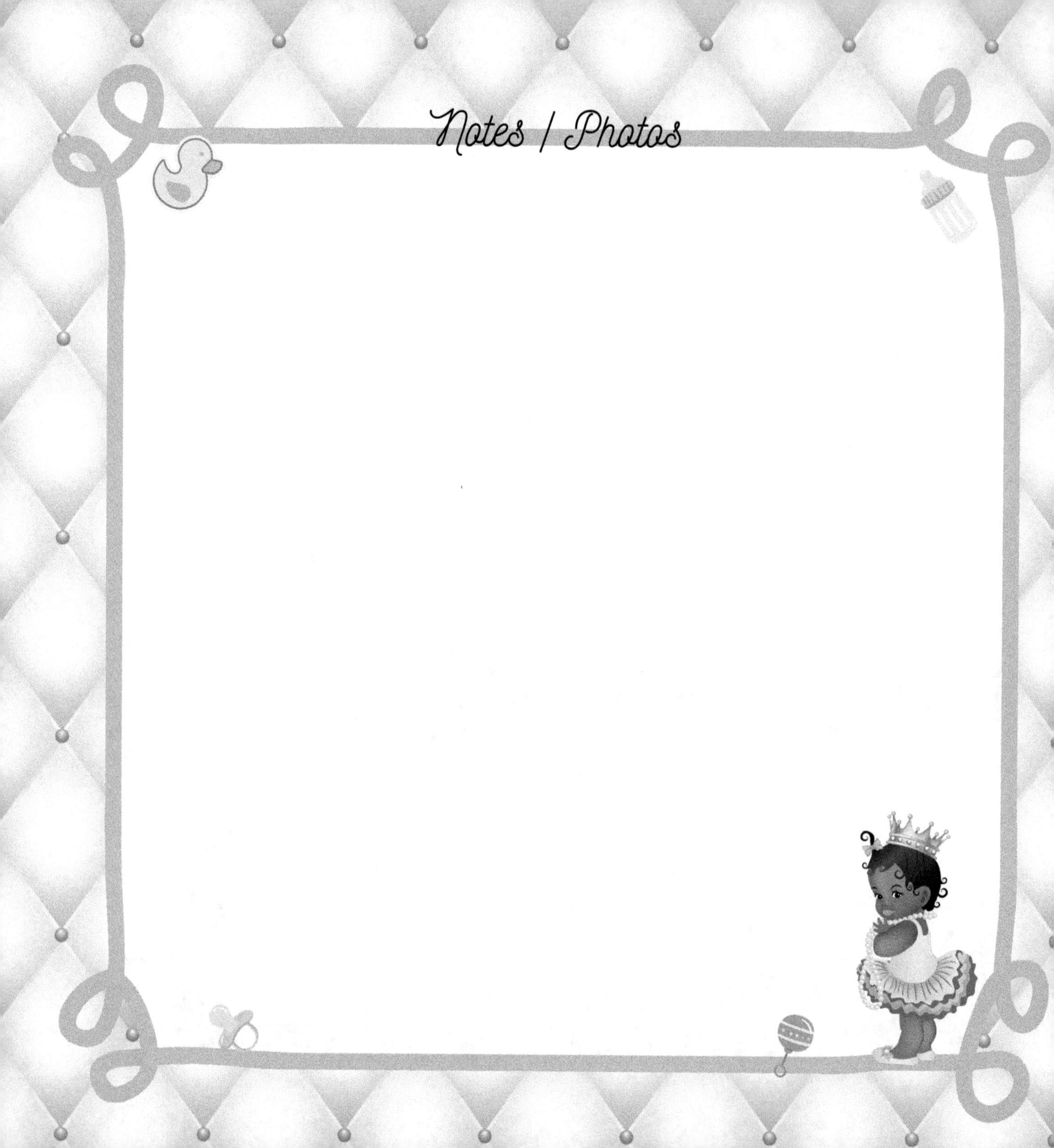

Notes / Photos

Notes / Photos

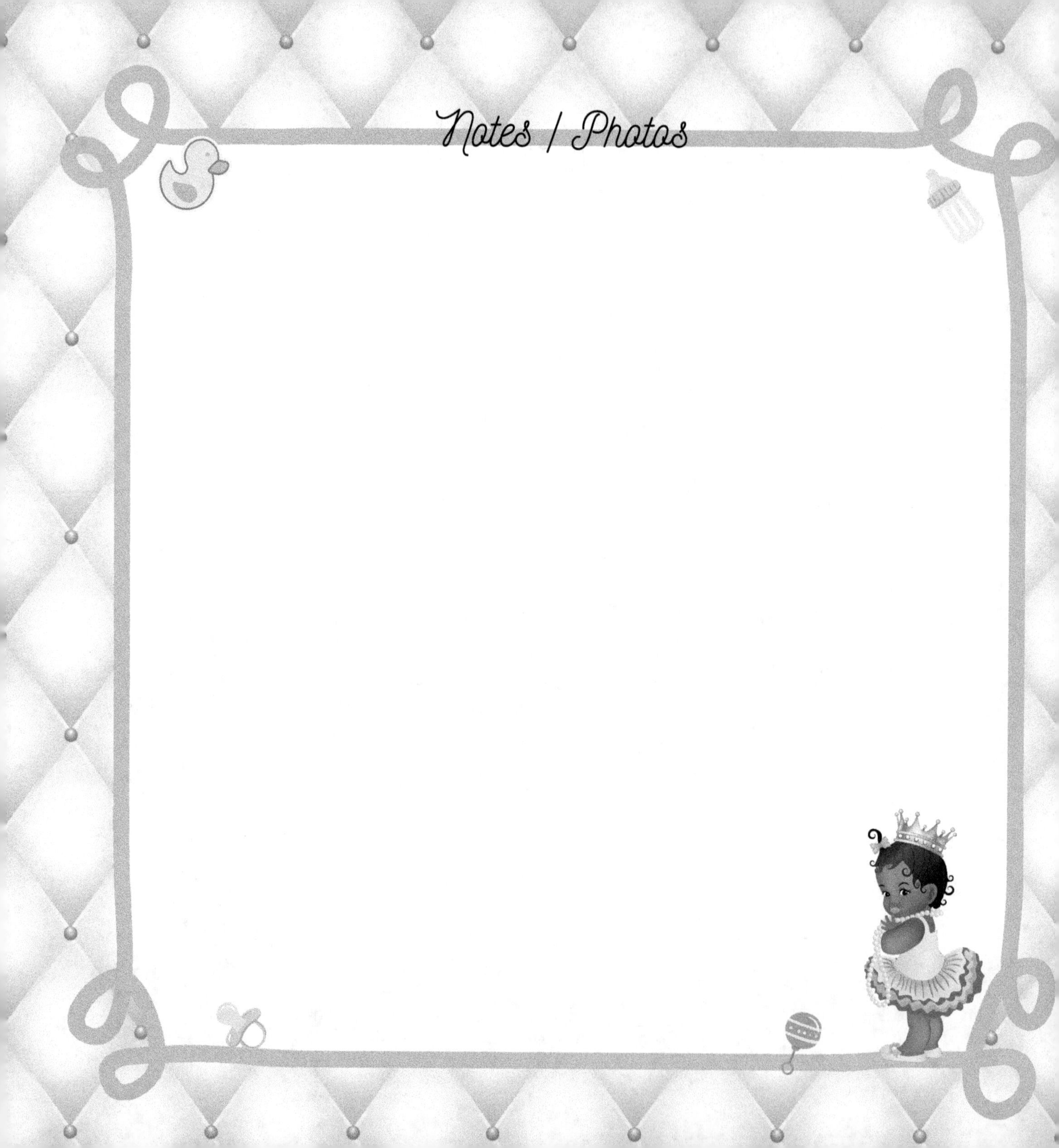

Notes / Photos

Notes / Photos

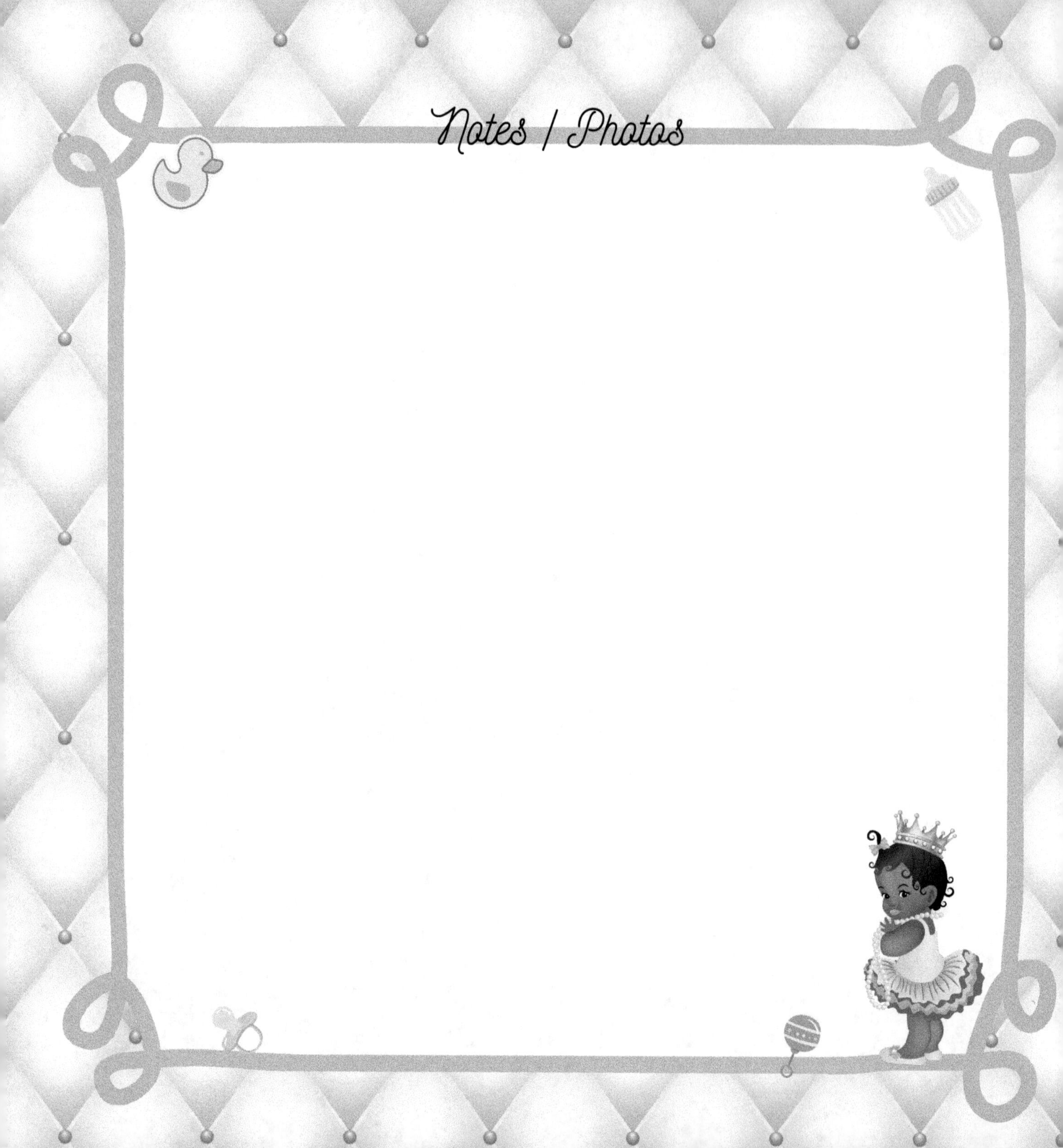

Notes / Photos

Gift Log

Name/Email/Phone

Gift

Gift Log

Name/Email/Phone | Gift

Gift Log

Name/Email/Phone   Gift

Gift Log

Name/Email/Phone	Gift

Gift Log

Name/Email/Phone | Gift

Gift Log

Name/Email/Phone	Gift

Gift Log

Name/Email/Phone   Gift

Gift Log

Name/Email/Phone   Gift

Gift Log

Name/Email/Phone   Gift

Gift Log

Name/Email/Phone   Gift